I'M IN YOUR VACCINES

This book will be slightly unconventional in its layout and fashion in which it unfolds. Mostly because, that's the point. Our lives unfold exactly like that, and this book will chronical much of how I arrived at my decisions in regards to vaccines when it comes to my family.

This book is in no way an attempt to tell you what to do, or shame you for anything you have done in the past. It is simply to inform you of the things that are deliberately kept from your sight and your decision making process because of the power the pharmaceutical company, and unfortunately our Government – has in the ability to sway the narrative in one direction or another (let's be real – it's just one direction).

Please do your best to follow along and really take the following points in for yourself, and understand that there will be cognitive dissonance in many places. Cognitive dissonance is simply the difficulty accepting new information when it directly contradicts what you believe to be true. This doesn't mean you're "dumb" – it simply means that changing our minds or looking at new information can be difficult. That's all. The more we are aware of it – the easier it is to overcome.

Let's start off with why this book even exists in the first place.

I was laying in bed after breaking my toe, stubbing it up a landmine my wife had so graciously left for me during the course of us getting ready to move south for the winter.

As I lay furious in bed about the hazards conveniently placed around the house, always in the middle of the room when there was BEYOND ample room for things to be moved into places that didn't resemble booby-traps for an unsuspecting husband with his contacts out, fumbling about like an ape in the dark – it apparently had turned out God had a plan for me to stub my toe and lay awake to get my wrath and fury under control so that He/She might intervene and say "I've got a mission for you".

I'm not saying I'm anything special – this is just how it happened and what inspired me to get cracking on this. Many times, it's in the bathtub or laying in bed unable to sleep when inspiration comes to me and I can say "Yes, I'll do this" or "No I'm going to be a lazy bum and ignore my intuition". I always try to choose the former.

As I laid and thought over ALL the things that I had to get into this book in a short amount of time, it of course was a bit daunting. However, after a little cursing my pulsing and throbbing toe, I figured there's no better place to start than the beginning and let the events and information unfold naturally, exactly how it did.

I suppose you could say I need simply tell the Truth – as best as one possibly can.

Before we get started into the actual information of the book, a little bit of a back story of myself is important. Not because I'M important, but because everything leading up to the release of this more-so is.

A simple Facebook search will yield many different things about myself. I'm a little bit out there. I have a lot of hobbies, interests, accomplishments, and even more mistakes that have been made in my life. The last statement is probably the Truest of them all – the amount of mistakes I've made and things I've done wrong (or at least could have done better) is fairly astounding.

I'm into quantum physics, anatomy and physiology, astrology, cosmology, classical physics, I've played piano for over 30 years (and this music is an interest), I've been an activist, a self-taught photographer, am teaching myself videography and video editing, I run 5 businesses (with at least 2 more planned). I study occult wisdom, the tarot, Jungian psychology, I love crystals and essential oils, I have 200 pounds of quartz crystal singing bowls I enjoy playing very much, I study crystallography, the nature of light and quantum entanglement, and have 3 other previously published books.

I'm learning Biblical Hebrew with my non-dominant hand for full brain unification, my talks with business partners involve tearing apart the human genome and pairing Bible verses, mythology, symbolism, hieroglyphics, epigenetics, anatomy and physiology, brain structure as it relates to ancient Egyptian "Gods", sacred geometry, mathematics and numbers, gematria, and other codes hidden in ancient wisdoms.

All that being said – I was also once a roughly 300 pound alcoholic that drank 2 pots of coffee per day, a gallon of diet coke, smoked 2 packs of cigarettes per day, and about a billion other self-destructive things.

I spent a year in Iraq, and I have very strong opinions about the military and "flag waving", and have seen the insanity first hand.

None of this is to attempt to "talk myself up" – but is instead to let you know if you search around you'll find an entire hodge-podge of things about me.

Anyone that wants to say "this" or "that" about me – it's most likely probably True. Or false. I don't know, don't care.

That, however – is not the point.

While so many things about ME might be true – this book in essence isn't about me, I'm simply giving you a short account of me so you can get a feel for the picture I'm about to paint for you, and see if there's any way you might be able to relate to me, or what led me onto the path of discovery about "actual informed consent" when it comes to vaccines.

No matter what is, or is not true about me – in the end makes no difference. The information that I'm bringing to you is what is of importance.

I only ask that you judge the information for what it is – either True, Untrue, or a mix of both. I'm going to attempt to keep it as polarized into black/white as possible so that it's very easy to say "True" or "Not True" for yourself.

All of this being said – let's get started.

My journey into the decision to vaccinate or not started roughly 5-6 years ago from the time of writing this when my wife and I decided I was finally adult enough to take care of a child.

Are any of us truly ready?

Well no.

But as I'd mentioned, a long period of my life was spent in "Adult Childhood" where my wife was very nearly my "caretaker" as I attempted to get my life together after a decade of being an irresponsible drunk.

As every good Father (I use the word "Father" and not "Dad" because there's a very big difference between the two) would try to do – I wanted to make sure I made the best decisions to be the best Father I possibly could be for my child-to-be.

Every Man and Father wants to do a good job raising a child – they want to care for their child in the best ways possible and try not to make any mistakes (full knowing they are going to, but try not to).

There's the obvious things parents do like "what kind of crib will be safe" and "what kind of car seat will be safe", "what food will the baby eat" and "what clothes are safe". The obvious list of what "should" and what "shouldn't" be done (within a budget normally as well) to ensure the best possible potential future for your child.

After running through the majority of the "standard checklist" (which I'll be honest was the task of my wife…) – I instead turned my attention to the medical aspect and navigating the medical world. For any topics including and outside of vaccines when it comes to navigating the medical world you may also look up a book a friend and I wrote called "So You're Going To Have a Baby" which is on Amazon.

Focusing simply on the vaccine decision aspect is the purpose of this book. I'm also not going to put a lot of "science" into it – because we can't move onto scientific arguments until we can get past some basic, common sense things. As many people already know – the "science" is horrendously skewed, but we'll get to that later.

One of the first things that happened to spark me upon my journey was a conversation with my Mother Teri.

A few years prior my sister had gotten a Gardasil Vaccine (this was essentially the catalyst for everything) and she had a "normal" reaction as the doctors said of collapsing into seizures immediately after getting it.

As my Mother and I conversed further – we stumbled across a now fairly well-known topic of "ear infections and vaccines". At an early point in my life, I started with chronic ear infections and ended up getting tubes in my ears twice. My Mother just happened to be combing through my medical records and noticed that my ear infections started within about 2 days of getting a round of vaccines. While many people could chalk this up to "coincidence" – it should be noted that ear infections are listed in the vaccine inserts (that are never given to you beforehand) as a possible outcome to vaccination.

And thus, the journey started toward Truth.

The CDC

The first place nearly every parent goes to look to see if "vaccines are safe and effective" is the most commonly used resource called the "CDC" or "Centers for Disease Control".

In a perfect world, this would be the place to go. A Government agency that is tasked with protecting children that does exactly that. However…we don't live in a perfect world, and as a parent having done the research – I can arrive at no other conclusion except the CDC does exactly the opposite of what they were tasked to do.

Let's dive in.

Bill Thompson
This topic I will focus on very little – as it is covered in my other book "So You're Going To Have a Baby" – and it's a bit further back in date. It's still absolutely relevant – but essentially, he is a whistleblower that reported that when the reports/research of Thimerosal (mercury) was causing neurological tics in children – he and other workers were instructed to have a "trash can party" in which all of the data was to be destroyed. If you Google up "The Simpsonwood Meeting" you may also look even further into the cover up that happened.

Like I'd said – I'm not going to focus on this as much as it's such a long topic, I simply encourage you to look into it for yourself.

Andrew Wakefield
Ahhhh the often touted "charlatan" who was "discredited" and lost his license. The latter half of the statement is true – but discredited, not even close.

It is important to note that Dr Wakefield never said, "vaccines cause autism". He simply released a paper showing autistic kids have this pattern of having messed up gut health (as he was a gastroenterologist).

11 or 12 other doctors signed off on the paper – and only he lost his license, because he was the only one to speak up.

I also will not spend much time on this topic because you can simply go watch the move "VAXXED" and watch the behind the scenes story to get the picture painted. Also, I won't focus on it much because it was quite some time ago, and we could get into many different arguments that will just take up too much time. I'm trying to keep this simple.

Onto the important things
Here now we move onto what can be talked about today when it comes to the irresponsibility of the CDC.

"Vaccine ingredients do not cause autism"
This is a multi-pronged statement that must be addressed in different parts.

The first part is that Thimerosal is safe and does not cause autism, and the CDC will list that they have 8 CDC FUNDED studies proving Thimerosal is safe, and you may head here to find them:
https://www.cdc.gov/vaccinesafety/concerns/autism.html

The only problem is, they list 8 studies that Thimerosal is safe. Only 8. If you still haven't looked up the Simpsonwood Meeting transcripts I encourage you to do so, but let's move onto simpler topics.

Thimerosal:
The ONLY study ever done on Thimerosal was done back around 1930 (give or take a few years) in which 27 meningitis patients were given Thimerosal as a "test" to see if it could be used as a treatment for meningitis.

EVERY. SINGLE. PATIENT. DIED.

This was their basis for proving "Thimerosal is safe" until people started to question it (especially after the Simpsonwood Meeting).

But let's just do this – let's look at the science today.

I encourage you to head to www.pubmed.gov and type in the words "Thimerosal Toxicity"

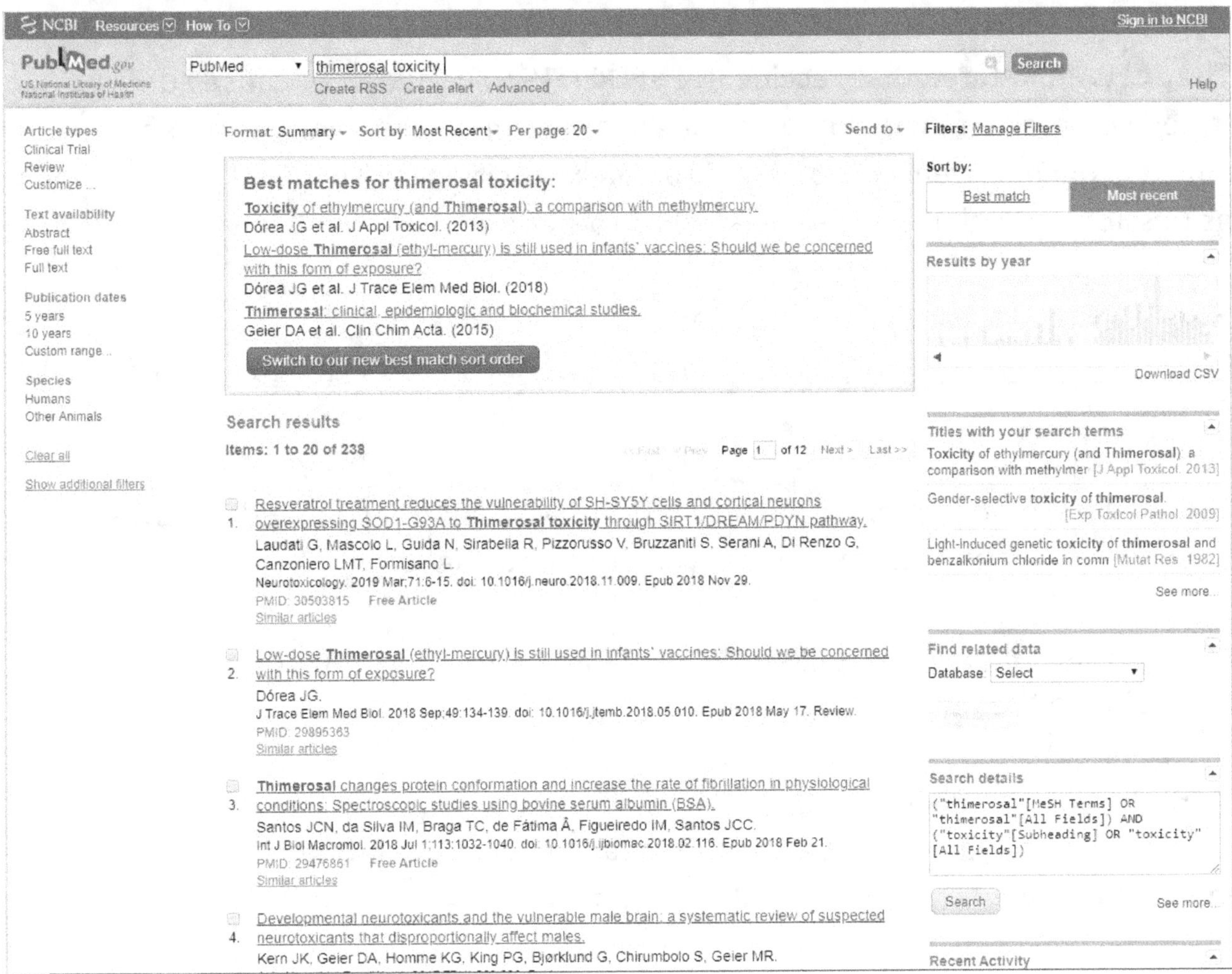

The search yields over 235 results, and if you're a responsible parent like myself, you comb through every article and see how many are relevant and are what you are looking for.

After combing through them – I found over 150 articles that stated BEYOND A DOUBT that Thimerosal was toxic in every way, shape, and form.

We don't have to sit and nit-pick apart all 8 studies from the CDC saying Thimerosal is safe, when we have over 20 times the studies saying Thimerosal is toxic. This is an example of the CDC "cherry picking" studies to cover its ass, you don't have to be a rocket scientist to put this together.

Now, what about the rest of the ingredients?

They CLEARLY stated that vaccine INGREDIENTS (plural) do not cause autism. When you click on their link to "what's in a vaccine" – they bring you to no other studies, and not even a list of what's actually in vaccines. They make it as generic as possible of "ohh it's just eggs or Jello" to stabilize it.

Here is instead the list you should read:
https://www.cdc.gov/vaccines/pubs/pinkbook/downloads/appendices/b/excipient-table-2.pdf

You'll notice how they don't publicly put this list right on the standard CDC site but you instead have to know what you are searching for.

Let's look at some of the "ingredients" that are "common and don't cause autism" according to the CDC:

-MRC-5 Cells and DNA
Also known as "Aborted Fetal Cells" – meaning an entire human genome is being injected into your child from an aborted fetus.

-FD&C Yellow #6 aluminum lake dye
So, you're saying my child isn't "yellow" enough and needs dyes injected into them?

-Monosodium Glutamate
I don't think I need to elaborate on how much research is out there that this can cause brain excitotoxicity issues

-Polysorbate 80
This is a product used to open the Blood Brain Barrier in animal experiments to allow different drugs and substances through it - which when injecting aluminum, which is a KNOW neurotoxin as an adjuvant, to "stimulate the immune system" –

what happens when the polysorbate 80 opens the blood brain barrier and the body is filled with "immune stimulating" neurotoxins? Babies already have under-developed blood brain barriers, why are we opening it more with polysorbate 80 (which is also in the Vitamin K shot – which carries a black box warning. See the book "So You're Going To Have a Baby" on Amazon for more)

-Bovine Fetal Serum

This is one of the best examples that I find as "interesting" as the aborted fetal cells being injected into a child, and is the reason for the book cover and title. One could probably confidently say – there's probably about 1% of doctors that have any idea this is an ingredient. But I digress – I'll wait for the "peer reviewed study" on how many doctors know this before I make any solid claims.

Vaccine Excipient Summary
Excipients Included in U.S. Vaccines, by Vaccine

In addition to weakened or killed disease antigens (viruses or bacteria), vaccines contain very small amounts of other ingredients – excipients.

Some excipients are added to a vaccine for a specific purpose. These include:
Preservatives, to prevent contamination. For example, thimerosal.
Adjuvants, to help stimulate a stronger immune response. For example, aluminum salts.
Stabilizers, to keep the vaccine potent during transportation and storage. For example, sugars or gelatin.

Others are residual trace amounts of materials that were used during the manufacturing process and removed. These can include:
Cell culture materials, used to grow the vaccine antigens. For example, egg protein, various culture media.
Inactivating ingredients, used to kill viruses or inactivate toxins. For example, formaldehyde.
Antibiotics, used to prevent contamination by bacteria. For example, neomycin.

The following table lists substances, other than active ingredients (i.e., antigens), shown in the manufacturers' package insert (PI) as being contained in the final formulation of each vaccine. **Note: Substances used in the manufacture of a vaccine but not listed as contained in the final product (e.g., culture media) can be found in each PI, but are not shown on this table.** Each PI, which can be found on the FDA's website (see below) contains a description of that vaccine's manufacturing process, including the amount and purpose of each substance. In most PIs, this information is found in Section 11: "Description."

All information was extracted from manufacturers' package inserts.
If in doubt about whether a PI has been updated since this table was prepared, check the FDA's website at:
http://www.fda.gov/BiologicsBloodVaccines/Vaccines/ApprovedProducts/ucm093833.htm

Vaccine	Contains
Adenovirus	monosodium glutamate, sucrose, D-mannose, D-fructose, dextrose, human serum albumin, potassium phosphate, plasdone C, anhydrous lactose, microcrystalline cellulose, polacrilin potassium, magnesium stearate, cellulose acetate phthalate, alcohol, acetone, castor oil, FD&C Yellow #6 aluminum lake dye
Anthrax (Biothrax)	aluminum hydroxide, sodium chloride, benzethonium chloride, formaldehyde
BCG (Tice)	glycerin, asparagine, citric acid, potassium phosphate, magnesium sulfate, iron ammonium citrate, lactose
Cholera (Vaxchora)	ascorbic acid, hydrolyzed casein, sodium chloride, sucrose, dried lactose, sodium bicarbonate, sodium carbonate
DT (Sanofi)	aluminum phosphate, isotonic sodium chloride, formaldehyde
DTaP (Daptacel)	aluminum phosphate, formaldehyde, glutaraldehyde, 2-phenoxyethanol
DTaP (Infanrix)	formaldehyde, aluminum hydroxide, sodium chloride, polysorbate 80 (Tween 80)
DTaP-IPV (Kinrix)	Formaldehyde, aluminum hydroxide, sodium chloride, polysorbate 80 (Tween 80), neomycin sulfate, polymyxin B
DTaP-IPV (Quadracel)	formaldehyde, aluminum phosphate, 2-phenoxyethanol, polysorbate 80, glutaraldehyde, neomycin, polymyxin B sulfate, bovine serum albumin
DTaP-HepB-IPV (Pediarix)	formaldehyde, aluminum hydroxide, aluminum phosphate, sodium chloride, polysorbate 80 (Tween 80), neomycin sulfate, polymyxin B, yeast protein
DTaP-IPV/Hib (Pentacel)	aluminum phosphate, polysorbate 80, sucrose, formaldehyde, glutaraldehyde, bovine serum albumin, 2-phenoxyethanol, neomycin, polymyxin B sulfate
Hib (ActHIB)	sodium chloride, formaldehyde, sucrose
Hib (Hiberix)	formaldehyde, sodium chloride, lactose
Hib (PedvaxHIB)	amorphous aluminum hydroxyphosphate sulfate, sodium chloride
Hep A (Havrix)	MRC-5 cellular proteins, formalin, aluminum hydroxide, amino acid supplement, phosphate-buffered saline solution, polysorbate 20, neomycin sulfate, aminoglycoside antibiotic
Hep A (Vaqta)	amorphous aluminum hydroxyphosphate sulfate, non-viral protein, DNA, bovine albumin, formaldehyde, neomycin, sodium borate, sodium chloride, other process chemical residuals
Hep B (Engerix-B)	aluminum hydroxide, yeast protein, sodium chloride, disodium phosphate dihydrate, sodium dihydrogen phosphate dihydrate
Hep B (Recombivax)	formaldehyde, potassium aluminum sulfate, amorphous aluminum hydroxyphosphate sulfate, yeast protein

You're an adult however and can go read them for yourself.

The biggest question to ask is…

If the CDC says "Vaccine Ingredients Do Not Cause Autism" – I simply ask them, well where are your studies showing injecting the **entire human genome** of another human being who was aborted into my child is safe? Don't you think the burden of the proof should be on them in this case?

Where are the studies showing all of these ingredients from up to 8 vaccines at once in one visit are safe? I mean – they said they don't cause autism….so, where is the proof?

And it's not just autism – the question begs what OTHER health problems could result from this?

I've read an insert – some have PAGES worth of paragraphs listing all the different adverse events that can occur, it's funny how all of that is neglected on the CDC's website.

"Vaccines do not cause autism"

This statement is directly at the CDC website here:
https://www.cdc.gov/vaccinesafety/concerns/autism.html

Here also you can download the exact same paper they have listed to see for yourself the exact words I will use in the next picture (so you don't have to believe me) – or simply click on their citation on their site:
http://nationalacademies.org/hmd/~/media/Files/Report%20Files/201
1/Adverse-Effects-of-Vaccines-Evidence-and-Causality/Vaccine-report-
brief-FINAL.pdf

Now, let's take a look at the highlighted section below in this picture, from their very paper:

Evidence Favors Acceptance of a Causal Relationship

The evidence favors acceptance of four vaccine–adverse event relationships. In these cases, the evidence is strong and generally suggestive, but not firm enough to be described as convincing. These relationships include:

- HPV vaccine and anaphylaxis;
- MMR vaccine and transient arthralgia (temporary joint pain) in female adults;
- MMR vaccine and transient arthralgia in children; and
- certain trivalent inactivated influenza vaccines used in Canada in some recent years and a mild and temporary oculorespiratory syndrome, which is characterized by conjunctivitis, facial swelling, and upper respiratory symptoms, including coughing and wheezing.

Evidence Favors Rejection of a Causal Relationship

The evidence favors rejection of five vaccine–adverse event relationships:

- MMR vaccine and autism
- MMR vaccine and type 1 diabetes
- DTaP (tetanus) vaccine and type 1 diabetes
- Inactivated influenza vaccine and Bell's palsy (weakness of the facial nerve)
- Inactivated influenza vaccine and exacerbation of asthma or reactive airway disease episodes in children and adults

Evidence Inadequate to Accept or Reject a Causal Relationship

For the vast majority, (135 vaccine-adverse event pairs), the evidence is inadequate to accept or reject a causal relationship. In many cases, the adverse event being examined is an extremely rare condition, making it hard to study. In these cases, there was not adequate evidence to determine if the vaccine was or was not causally associated.

Not the very words on the CDC's own site:
"Vaccine**S** (plural) do not cause autism"

However – when looking at the one study they used to back up their statement....only one vaccine, by itself, according to them, does not cause autism.

So...WHERE did they get the information to state vaccines *PLURAL* or in combination do not cause autism? How did they arrive at that conclusion?

Simply put – they have absolutely no data to back that up. Their own data says so itself that ONLY the MMR vaccine on its OWN doesn't cause autism.

We could go through and scientifically argue whether ONE study is enough to prove that vaccines do or don't cause autism – but that's not the point I'm trying to make.

The POINT is that there is not ONE study that they have to support their statement that vaccines PLURAL – as in ALL the vaccines have been studied as to whether they cause autism or not – DOES NOT EXIST. I'm using their paper and saying what they have said in their study is True. I'm not even arguing to discredit their science. I'm simply pointing out that they do not have ANY evidence that vaccines PLURAL (either alone or in combination)do not cause autism based on their own studies to justify it.

The point I'm trying to make here – is that it is utterly RECKLESS and IRRESPONSIBLE to tell parents "Vaccines (PLURAL) do not cause autism" because their one study said one vaccine by itself does not cause autism.

What about all the other vaccines? What about giving more than vaccine at once?

This leads me to my next point.

Not one study shows that the current vaccine schedule is safe or that giving more than one vaccine at once is safe

After I'd discovered this, I like a logical person started to doubt and question the things I'd been told and not take them at face value. ESPECIALLY when to make such a ludicrous statement based on very obvious data and facts would be so RECKLESS and IRRESPONSIBLE.

So, I decided to go a step further.

I myself emailed the CDC and asked two questions:
"Do you have any studies showing the current CDC vaccine schedule is safe?"
"Do you have any studies showing that giving more than one vaccine at once is safe?"

Their response back was nothing short of astounding.

In regards to the first question – not one piece of data they could provide me could show that the current vaccine schedule is safe. They sent me different studies and links that assured me "vaccines are safe and effective" – but could not link me to ONE study that compared unvaccinated or less vaccinated children against fully vaccinated according to their schedule. We will come back to this again shortly.

"Do you have any studies showing that giving more than one vaccine at once is safe?"

Their response did not compare any mortality rates or illness rates against children receiving more than one vaccine at once to those who got only one. The only thing they sent me was a study showing more antigens being added into a single vaccine proved to be safe.

I told them "this is not what I asked for – I asked for studies on MULTIPLE vaccines at once being given is safe".

They simply responded to "stop emailing them and fill out an Freedom of Information Request" in regards to this matter.

Don't take my word for it though – email them yourself and ask for the studies that giving more than one vaccine at once is safe.

See what you get.

Here is my simple rebuttal to it – a scientific article published in "Journal of American Physicians and Surgeons" magazine, which you may view yourself here: http://vaccinesafetycommission.org/pdfs/04-2016-JPANDS-Miller-Vaccines.pdf

You can download it in dozens of places if you want to search for it yourself, but let's look at the conclusion the ONLY scientific paper to be done on this found below:

significant 50% higher mortality rate compared with those who had received fewer.

The Age Effect on Hospitalizations and Death

Our study also analyzed whether the age at which an infant received vaccines had an effect on hospitalizations and death. Of the 38,801 VAERS reports that we analyzed, 765 concerned infants six-weeks-old or younger who received one or more vaccine doses prior to the adverse event, and 154 of those infants were hospitalized: a hospitalization rate of 20.1%. Of 5,572 infants aged six months at vaccination, 858 were hospitalized: 15.4%. Of 801 infants who were nearly a year old when they were vaccinated, 86 were hospitalized: 10.7%. The hospitalization rate decreased linearly from 20.1% for neonates to 10.7% for older infants. Linear regression analysis of hospitalization rates as a function of patient age yielded an R^2 of 0.95.

In the 38,801 VAERS reports we analyzed, 26,408 infants were younger than six months. After receiving one or more vaccine doses, 1,623 of those infants died: a mortality rate of 6.1%. The remaining 12,393 infants were between six months and one year of age. After receiving one or more vaccine doses, 258 of them died: 2.1%. The mortality rate for vaccinated infants younger than six months was significantly higher than the mortality rate for vaccinated infants aged between six months and one year, with an RR = 3.0 (95% CI, 2.6-3.4). Infants who had an adverse event reported to VAERS were significantly more likely to be hospitalized or die if they were younger rather than older at the time of vaccination.

Summary of Results and Media Response

Our study showed that infants who receive several vaccines concurrently, as recommended by CDC, are significantly more likely to be hospitalized or die when compared with infants who receive fewer vaccines simultaneously. It also showed that reported adverse effects were more likely to lead to hospitalization or death in younger infants.

These findings are so troubling that we expected major media outlets in America to sound an alarm, calling for an immediate reevaluation of current preventive health care practices. But 4 years after publication of our study, this has not happened. Could it be because, according to Robert Kennedy, Jr., about 70% of advertising revenue on network news comes from drug companies? In fact, the president of a network news division admitted that he would fire a host who brought on a guest that led to loss of a pharmaceutical account. That may be why the mainstream media won't give equal time to stories about problems with vaccine safety.[15]

Conclusion

The safety of CDC's childhood vaccination schedule was never affirmed in clinical studies. Vaccines are administered to millions of infants every year, yet health authorities have no scientific data from synergistic toxicity studies on all combinations of vaccines that infants are likely to receive. National vaccination campaigns must be supported by scientific evidence. No child should be subjected to a health policy that is not based on sound scientific principles and, in fact, has been shown to be potentially dangerous.

pharmaceutical advertising revenue to change their business models so that crucial scientific research, regardless of how controversial it may be, is widely disseminated into the public domain. Meanwhile, the evidence presented in this study shows that multiple vaccines administered during one visit, and vaccinating young infants, significantly increase morbidity and mortality. Parents and physicians should consider health options associated with a lower risk of hospitalization or death.

Neil Z. Miller is a medical research journalist. Contact: neilzmiller@gmail.com.

Disclosures: No conflicts of interest were disclosed.

REFERENCES

1. U.S. Department of Health and Human Services. National Vaccine Injury Compensation Program. Available at: http://www.hrsa.gov/vaccinecompensation. Accessed Feb 14, 2016.
2. U.S. Department of Health and Human Services. Vaccine Adverse Event Reporting System (VAERS). Available at: https://vaers.hhs.gov. Accessed Feb 14, 2016.
3. Institute of Medicine (U.S.) Vaccine Safety Committee. Appendix B: Strategies for Gathering Information. In: *Adverse Events Associated with Childhood Vaccines: Evidence Bearing on Causality.* Stratton KR, Howe CJ, Johnston RB Jr., eds. Washington, D.C.: National Academies Press (U.S.); 1994. Available at: http://www.ncbi.nlm.nih.gov/books/NBK236281. Accessed Mar 5, 2016.
4. Sukumaran L, McNeil MM, Moro PL, et al. Adverse events following measles, mumps, and rubella vaccine in adults reported to the Vaccine Adverse Event Reporting System (VAERS), 2003-2013. *Clin Infect Dis* 2015;60(10):e58-65.
5. Haber P, Moro PL, McNeil MM, et al. Post-licensure surveillance of trivalent live attenuated influenza vaccine in adults, United States, Vaccine Adverse Event Reporting System (VAERS), July 2005-June 2013. *Vaccine* 2014;32(48):6499-6504.
6. Haber P, Patel M, Pan Y, et al. Intussusception after rotavirus vaccines reported to U.S. VAERS, 2006-2012. *Pediatrics* 2013;131(6):1042-1049.
7. Geier DA, Hooker BS, Kern JK, et al. A two-phase study evaluating the relationship between thimerosal-containing vaccine administration and the risk for an autism spectrum disorder diagnosis in the United States. *Transl Neurodegener* 2013;2(1):25.
8. Geier DA, Kern JK, King PG, Sykes LK, Geier MR. The risk of neurodevelopmental disorders following a thimerosal-preserved DTaP formulation in comparison to its thimerosal-reduced formulation in the Vaccine Adverse Event Reporting System (VAERS). *J Biochem Pharmacol Res* 2014;2(2):64-73.
9. Geier DA, Geier MR. An assessment of the impact of thimerosal on childhood neurodevelopmental disorders. *Pediatr Rehabil* 2003;6(2):97-102.
10. Lai YC, Yew YW. Severe autoimmune adverse events post *Herpes zoster* vaccine: a case-control study of adverse events in a national database. *J Drugs Dermatol* 2015;14(7):681-684.
11. Miller NZ. *Miller's Review of Critical Vaccine Studies: 400 Important Scientific Papers Summarized for Parents and Researchers.* Santa Fe, N.M.: New Atlantean Press; 2016.
12. Castranova V, Graham J, Hearl F, et al. Mixed exposures research agenda: a report by the NORA Mixed Exposures Team. Department of Health and Human Services (DHHS), Centers for Disease Control and Prevention (CDC), National Institute for Occupational Safety and Health (NIOSH). DHHS (NIOSH) Publication No. 2005-106; December 2004:vi. Available at: http://www.cdc.gov/niosh/docs/2005-106/pdfs/2005-106.pdf. Accessed Feb 14, 2016.
13. Offit PA, Quarles J, Gerber MA, et al. Addressing parents' concerns: do multiple vaccines overwhelm or weaken the infant's immune system? *Pediatrics* 2002;109(1):124-129.
14. Goldman GS, Miller NZ. Relative trends in hospitalizations and mortality among infants by the number of vaccine doses and age, based on the Vaccine Adverse Event Reporting System (VAERS), 1990-2010. *Hum Exp Toxicol* 2012;31(10):1012-1021. Available at: http://het.sagepub.com/content/31/10/1012.full. Accessed Feb 14, 2016.
15. Jaxen, J. Kennedy drops bombshell: 70% news ad revenue from pharma. *Before It's News*, May 22, 2015. Available at: http://beforeitsnews.com/health/2015/05/kennedy-drops-bombshell-70-news-ad-revenue-from-pharma-2574590.html. Accessed Feb 14, 2016.

18

For those that have trouble reading it you may read the summary of results here:

"Our study showed that infants who receive several vaccines concurrently, as recommended by CDC, are significantly more likely to be hospitalized or die when compared with infants who receive fewer vaccines simultaneously. It also showed that reported adverse effects were more likely to lead to hospitalization or death in younger infants."

This was the study I had emailed to the CDC asking if they had anything that would speak against it. I don't want to rely on just ONE study if I don't have to – but unfortunately I have not been able to find anything else that very simply breaks down the mortality and injury rate of children receiving none or just one vaccine in comparison to multiple.

By all means though – email them yourself and ask if they have such a study to counter this one. As a parent – if the CDC is going to tell you how safe vaccines are, it should be very easy to produce a number of studies to back up your claims that provide direct contrary evidence to this one.

Multiple Vaccines and SIDS

Since we're on this topic of multiple vaccines at once, there is another study I happened across in my research that is extremely relevant here.

The United States has the highest infant mortality rate of any 1st world, and even some 2nd world countries.

If we spend more on healthcare than basically the rest of the world combined, and give more "life saving vaccines" than any other country...why is our infant mortality rate the WORST of any first world country?

A 30 second Google search will confirm this statement of our mortality rates – go have a peek for yourself.

This then leads me to the topic of SIDS. "Death" is listed in EVERY vaccine insert as a potential outcome of vaccination. Do we know the ACTUAL numbers of how many people ACTUALLY die from vaccines?

No, because we use a passive system known as VAERS which I will address later. For now let's look at this interesting research article:

https://academic.oup.com/cid/article/61/6/980/451431?fbclid=IwAR1HTkIXRIBm G2auhtqjg3Jmg70YBKcHVzp8bIsWI-U-iafIUlggRuTMqJk

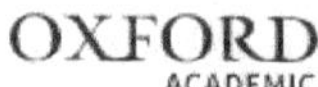

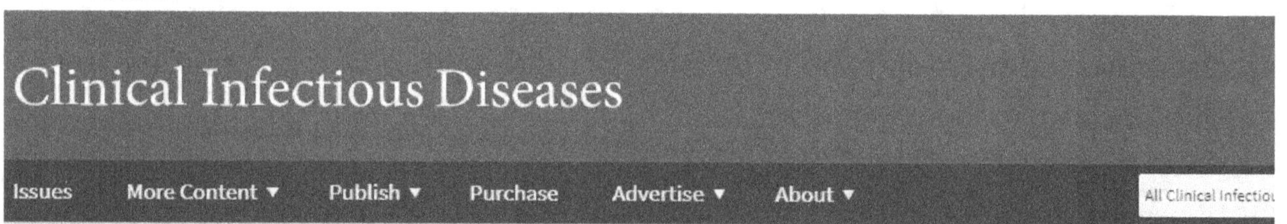

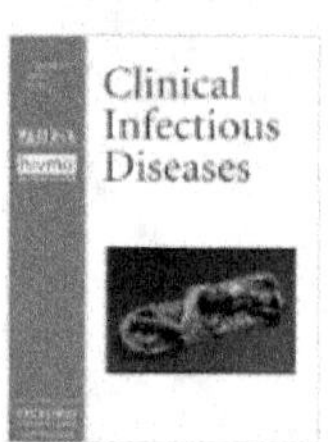

Volume 61, Issue 6
15 September 2015

Article Contents

Abstract

METHODS

RESULTS

DISCUSSION

Notes

References

💬 Comments (0)

< Previous   Next >

EDITOR'S CHOICE

Deaths Reported to the Vaccine Adverse Event Reporting System, United States, 1997–2013 🆓

Pedro L. Moro ✉, Jorge Arana, Maria Cano, Paige Lewis, Tom T. Shimabukuro

Clinical Infectious Diseases, Volume 61, Issue 6, 15 September 2015, Pages 980–987, https://doi.org/10.1093/cid/civ423
Published: 28 May 2015   Article history ▼

🅐 PDF   ❚❚ Split View   ❝❝ Cite   🔑 Permissions   ❮ Share ▼

Abstract

Background.   Vaccines are among the safest medical products in use today. Hundreds of millions of vaccinations are administered in the United States each year. Serious adverse reactions are uncommon. However, temporally associated deaths can occur following vaccination. Our aim was to characterize main causes of death among reports submitted to the US Vaccine Adverse Event Reporting System (VAERS), a spontaneous vaccine safety surveillance system.

Methods.   We searched VAERS for US reports of death after any vaccination from 1 July 1997 through 31 December 2013. Available medical records, autopsy reports, and death certificates were reviewed to identify cause of death.

Results.   VAERS received 2149 death reports, most (n = 1469 [68.4%]) in children. Median age was 0.5 years (range, 0–100 years); males accounted for 1226 (57%) reports. The total annual number of death reports generally decreased during the latter part of the study period. Most common causes of death among 1244 child reports with available death certificates/autopsy

Now, let's zoom in just a little closer…

79.4% of infants who died in their first year had one or more vaccines within 24 hours of death.

It does not take a rocket scientist to say "wait a second, how did nearly 80% of children who mysteriously died have one or more vaccines within 24 hours of death?"

If I were to take a bunch of kids – and 80% of them died mysteriously within 24 hours of me giving them Frankincense oil, you can sure as hell bet people would say "wait a second…." And there would be a gigantic uproar across all of America and the crackdown on Essential Oils would happen overnight.

Now however, I want to point out an even more disturbing part of this article:

"Conclusions.   No concerning pattern was noted among death reports submitted to VAERS during 1997–2013. The main causes of death were consistent with the most common causes of death in the US population.

Wait, what???

80% of all mysterious and unexplained deaths of children were within 24 hours of a vaccine, and this isn't a concerning pattern???

Ohh but we're not done yet either.

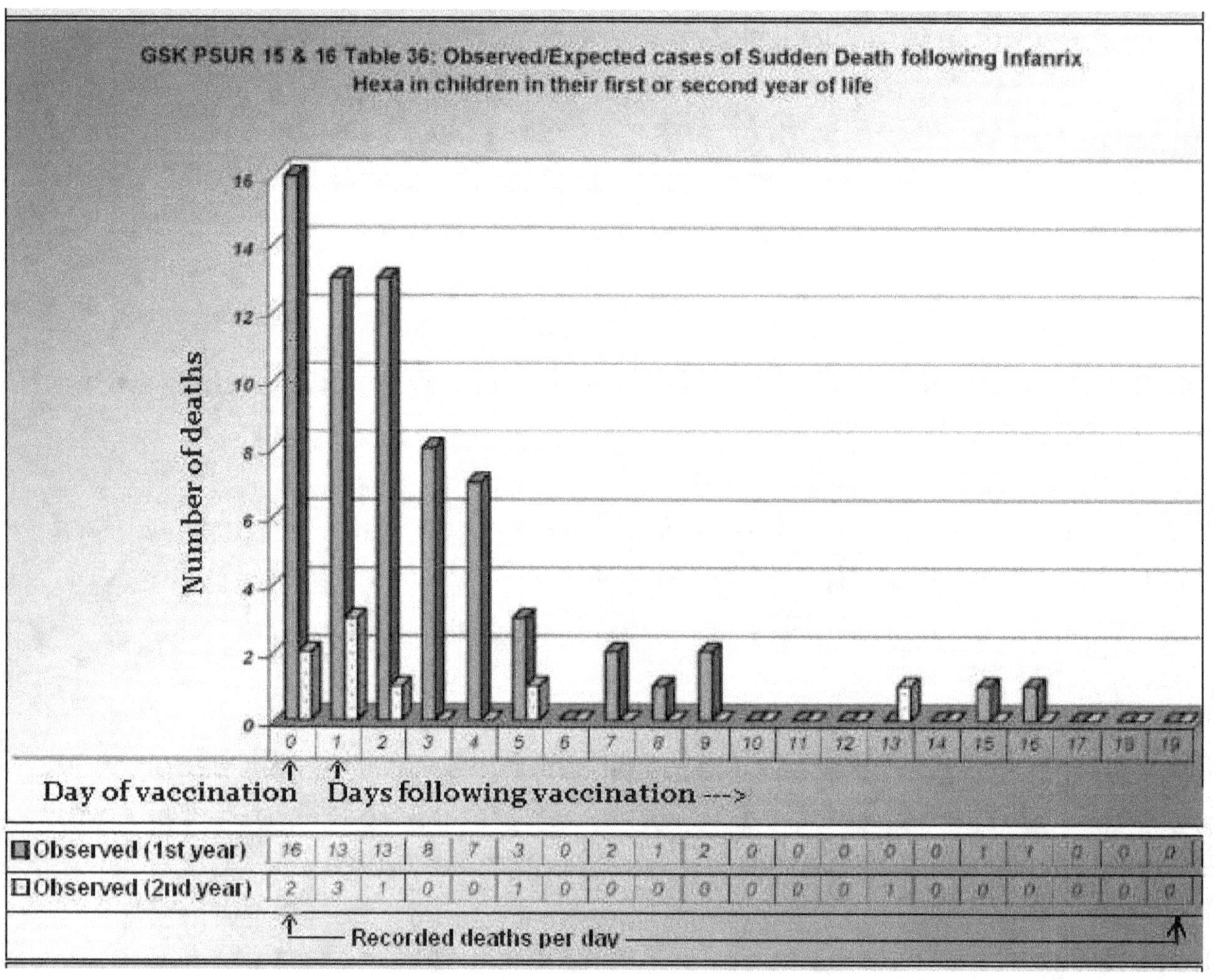

	0	1	2	3	4	5	6	7	8	9	10	11	12	13	14	15	16	17	18	19
Observed (1st year)	16	13	13	8	7	3	0	2	1	2	0	0	0	0	0	1	1	0	0	0
Observed (2nd year)	2	3	1	0	0	1	0	0	0	0	0	0	0	1	0	0	0	0	0	0

Here is a graph from the Infanrix – Glaxo Smith Kline's 6 in 1 vaccine – vaccine insert from their OWN data from clinical trials.

Notice how 90% of deaths in the approval trials are within the first 4 days after vaccination? This is THEIR OWN DATA!!!

Take ANY OTHER PRODUCT in the world – and produce a graph like this. Would you not take pause and say "wait – why are all the deaths clustered around the time we gave the kids said product?"

VAERS

Since we're on the topic of VAERS and deaths and reporting – let's talk about ANOTHER interesting fact that has recently surfaced.

It's a story about finding a better way to track vaccine injuries…

VAERS stands for Vaccine Adverse Events Reporting System – or more simply put, a way to track vaccine reactions after they are given. Call it a "poor man's post marketing tracking system".

Here's the problem though – the system is VOLUNTARY. Meaning – no one is REQUIRED to report vaccine adverse events into it.

The biggest problems here are that:

1.) Most doctors don't know how to identify an "adverse event" or reaction to a vaccine because they don't read the inserts, and believe "vaccines are safe and effective".
2.) Filling out a VAERS report is time consuming, and makes the doctors nothing – so there is less than NO incentive to do so.

Name the last time your doctor filled out a VAERS report for your sore arm, or when you got "the pretend flu" after getting a flu shot and you were miserable for days. Doesn't happen – because the system is set up to fail.

This means that roughly 1% of all vaccine reactions are actually reported – meaning the "1 in a million" vaccine reactions is nothing more than a slogan, it has no actual bearing on reality.

You can read all about the problems with VAERS from the CDC themselves here: https://www.cdc.gov/mmwr/preview/mmwrhtml/ss5201a1.htm

But let's use some actual data to see what happened when someone tried to make a better system.
First off here's the link to read everything for yourself I'm about to tell you:
https://truthsnitch.com/2017/10/24/cdc-silence-million-dollar-harvard-project-charged-upgrading-vaccine-safety-surveillance-system/#sthash.cDNk7FUm.dpbs

Here's an excerpt from it:

The Department of Health and Human Services (HHS) gave Harvard Medical School a <u>$1 million dollar grant</u> to track VAERS reporting at Harvard Pilgrim Healthcare for 3 years and to create an automated reporting system which would revolutionize the VAERS reporting system- transforming it from "passive" to "active."

This project was called Electronic Support for Public Heath- Vaccine Adverse Reporting System (ESPH:VAERS). According to the <u>grant final report</u>, the scope of the project was, "To create a generalizable system to facilitate detection and clinician reporting of vaccine adverse events, in order to improve the safety of national vaccination programs." To accomplish this the team used the electronic medical records at Harvard Pilgrim Healthcare, Inc, which is described as a "large multi-specialty practice." Every patient that received a vaccine was automatically identified and followed for 30 days. Within that 30 days the individual's diagnostic health codes, lab tests, and prescriptions were evaluated to recognize any potential adverse event. Another goal of the project was to evaluate the performance of the new automated system via a randomized trial and to compare this new data to the existing data collected by VAERS and Vaccine Safety Datalink.

Just the preliminary description of this program is head and shoulders above the current functioning of the passive VAERS system. In our current system, adverse events are to be spontaneously reported by parents or health care providers. Most parents aren't even aware the VAERS system exists, much less aware that they are supposed to be reporting to it. Health care providers are "supposed" to report adverse events, but we have no idea of the efficiency level with which this is occurring, and more than a hunch that this reporting is grossly neglected for a variety of reasons. Furthermore, many vaccine adverse events are never reported because either the parent, patient, or doctor is completely unaware that a subsequent adverse event is in fact due to a vaccine. This new reporting system would remove all of these failures from the equation.

What were the results?

Data was collected from June 2006 to October of 2009 on a total of 715,000 patients. Of those 715,000 patients, 376,452 were given 1.4 million doses of 45 different vaccines. A total of 35,570 possible adverse reactions were identified, so 2.6% of vaccinations were followed by a possible adverse reaction.

Let's just take a minute to reflect on that last sentence. Out of only 376,452 individuals that received a vaccine at this Harvard practice, the new automated system identified 35,570 possible adverse reactions in a three year period. How does that stack up to the number of adverse effects reported to VAERS? According to the CDC, only 30,000 adverse events are reported every year for the entire US population.

I'll quote the findings directly from the report, "Adverse events from drugs and vaccines are common, but underreported. [...] Likewise, fewer than 1% of vaccine adverse events are reported. Low reporting rates preclude or slow the identification of 'problem' drugs and vaccines that endanger public health. New surveillance methods for drug and vaccine adverse effects are needed."

Again, let's stop and think about this revelation for a moment - fewer than 1% of vaccine adverse events are reported. The CDC's entire vaccination propaganda campaign rests on their claim that side effects from vaccination are exceedingly rare (and predominantly minor).

According to the CDC, in 2016 alone, VAERS received 59,117 vaccine adverse event reports. Among those reports were 432 deaths, 1,091 permanent disabilities, 4,132 hospitalizations, and 10,274 emergency room visits. What if these numbers actually represent less than 1% of the total as this report asserts? Simple multiplication would yield vaccine adverse events reports numbering 5,911,700!

What was the CDC's response?

Basically, the same response your average college student falls back on when they decide they are no longer interested in continuing a relationship - they cut all lines of communication. No more answering phone calls or emails. You heard me correctly, the Centers for Disease Control **GHOSTED** Harvard Pilgrim Healthcare, Inc.

For those who are unaware, <u>Google dictionary</u> defines ghosting as, "the practice of ending a personal relationship by suddenly and without explanation withdrawing from all communication." Personally, I would hope that I could hold an organization like the CDC to a higher standard, but…

After a one million dollar grant was paid and three years of research conducted on what appeared to be a very successful upgrade to the passive VAERS system, the team's CDC contacts went MIA.

The ESPH - VAERS final report states, "Unfortunately, there was never an opportunity to perform system performance assessments because the necessary CDC contacts were no longer available and the CDC consultants responsible for receiving data were no longer responsive to our multiple requests to proceed with testing and evaluation."

According to the final report, the only thing left for the CDC to do was link the VAERS system to the Harvard Pilgrim system in order to transmit the data. The team requested that the CDC do this, "However, real data transmissions of non-physician approved reports to the CDC was unable to commence, as by the end of this project, the CDC had yet to respond to multiple requests to partner for this activity."

LET THAT SINK IN…

After spending A MILLION DOLLARS to improve vaccine adverse events reporting…

THE CDC SIMPLY STOPPED RESPONDING TO ANY AND ALL EMAILS AND CALLS

Ohh – but we're not done yet.

Let's talk about yet ANOTHER topic that is well hidden from the public's knowledge.

Glyphosate/Weedkiller contamination in vaccines

This is a topic that is near and dear to my heart – as I personally dealt with the FDA and their ability to completely disregard all common sense on this one.

On August 31, 2016 – the fine people at Moms Across America following a congressional hearing on RoundUp/Weedkiller being found in vaccines, sent a letter to numerous health agencies asking them to address the issue of vaccine contamination.

You may read a copy of the letter here:
https://d3n8a8pro7vhmx.cloudfront.net/yesmaam/pages/1707/attachments/orig inal/1473090145/LettertoFDACDCandCongressReVanccinesandGlyphosate_(1).pd f?1473090145

The tests were conducted with the Elisa method, which is regarded by the scientific community as a screening method only and not as accurate as HPLC mass spectrometry. Honeycutt reports that they asked numerous labs to test additional vaccines for glyphosate over the past few months and they have been unable to test. After learning of MAA's results, an independent scientist conducted numerous rounds of testing and has confirmed the presence of glyphosate in vaccines. He sent his data to Senator Sheehan, the FDA, NIH, elected government officials, major media, last week and received no response. One can contact **Senator Sheehan** for the additional test results.

Upon myself hearing said contamination (as this was over 3 years ago now) I personally called the FDA to ask if they were aware of the contamination and planned to do anything about it.

The first individual that I spoke with – merely hung up on the phone on me. Might have been because I was a bit "too outraged" about the fact that children were being pumped full of weedkiller via injections.

The next lady however was far more polite, and directed me to fill out an FOAI request in order to get the "official response" from the FDA – as she wasn't allowed to really comment on it.

She had let me know that they were indeed aware of it. So I asked "Well, does the FDA plan to do any testing to disprove it or address it?". Her response was "Well, no – what do you want vaccines to cost $1 Million Dollars apiece?".

So…she had let me know they knew about the contamination, were aware that it was true, but had no plans to do anything about it.

You may read the full story here:
https://www.momsacrossamerica.com/glyphosate_in_childhood_vaccines

So now, let's fast forward about 3 years.

The FDA and CDC in collusion FULL WELL KNOWING about the contamination of vaccines with weedkiller – kept it to themselves and decided NOT to let the public know about it.

When the FOAI request was submitted and the amount of time needed for the information to get out and get an "official" response from the FDA and the CDC about the contamination in vaccines – here is what happened.

"Yesterday, I received a letter from the CDC saying that we are giving you the information that we got from the FDA. I got fifty six pages; FIFTY SIX PAGES. It says some pages contain records that originated with the FDA, and are obscured. After careful review of these pages, some information was withheld from a release pursuant to five USC 522 exemption. So, what does that exemption look like? Blank pages! Every once in a while, we see an email saying "We need to respond to this, what do we say?" And then, more blank pages...more blank pages! What is the FDA hiding? What did they say? Why are they doing this?"

50% of the pages were completely blank or blacked out regarding the topic of weedkiller in vaccines!!!

Can you imagine this?

They simply "omitted" 50% of their conversations and findings regarding weedkiller being found in vaccines!!!

Does THIS sound like the wellbeing of your children is at the top of their "to-do" list???

Read the full article and review the blacked-out redacted response here: https://www.momsacrossamerica.com/fda_hides_information_on_glyphosate_in _vaccines

Cool news – we're STILL just getting started!!!

ICAN's lawsuit and FOAI to the DHHS regarding vaccine safety testing

Del Bigtree and Robert Kennedy Jr ended up filing a number of lawsuits against the US Government regarding vaccines and safety testing.

As it turns out – after the 1986 law that made vaccine manufacturers immune to lawsuits, the Department of Health and Human Services was tasked with reviewing vaccine safety every 2 years as part of the legal agreement in order to grant vaccine manufactures immunity to lawsuits regarding their products (vaccines).

If you didn't already know that vaccine manufacturers were immune to lawsuits regarding their products….well now you do. Anyhow, back to the subject…

After months of harassing the DHHS – Del, Robert, and the ICAN network ended up having to file a FOIA request, a Freedom Of Information Act request, along with filing a lawsuit in order to get the safety studies that the DHHS was supposed to be doing for the last 30 years.

Finally – months later, the DHS was finally forced to admit…..

IT HADN'T DONE A SINGLE SAFETY STUDY IN 30 YEARS.

You literally can't make this s*** up.

Ready for more…..?

Vaccines are not true placebo tested before release to market

 Del Bigtree and his team at ICAN released a stunning 88 page letter to the HHS regarding vaccine safety.

The letter, in response to an earlier reply from the then acting Director National Vaccine Program Office, Melinda Wharton, took virtually a year to compile, and is a meticulous piece of research.

Most sensationally they researched the HHS claim through US government archives that at least some pediatric vaccines had been trialed against genuine placebos, and came to a negative conclusion. Not only that, they established that none of the vaccines those vaccines had been trialed against had ever been trialed against genuine placebo either.

At the end of the line the toxic products were only being compared with other toxic products, rather than against saline.

Read the entire lawsuit and see all the data for yourself here:
https://www.icandecide.org/wp-content/uploads/2019/09/ICAN-Reply-1.pdf?fbclid=IwAR0lkZF2HV-AE3NIHgWyd5D1VAw1B11U2wFvaYOfLH9GUZm57pe0nQzMjSE

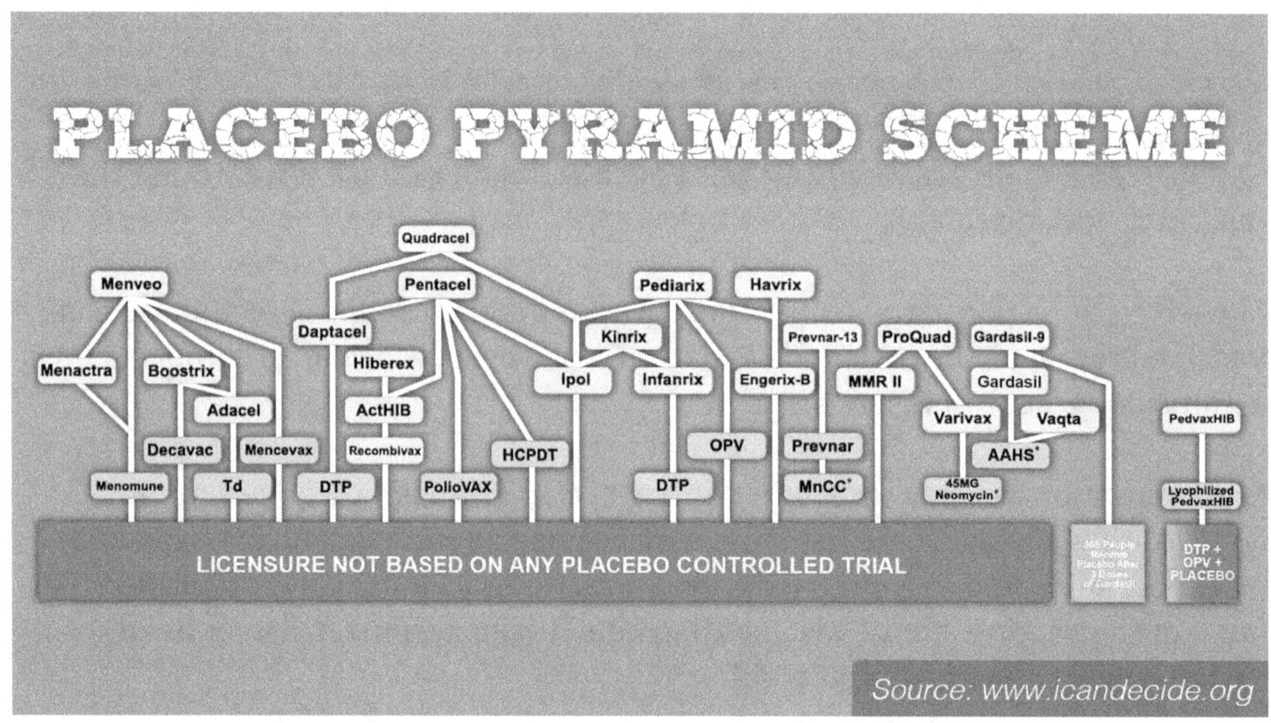

Parents, Mothers, Fathers – can you IMAGINE for ONE MOMENT, that a product immune to liability from lawsuits, has NEVER ONCE been tested against a true placebo?

Please, as a rational person – ask WHY on EARTH, if your product was SO GREAT – would you NOT test it against a true placebo???

I can give you a hint:

If you test poison against a true placebo – you'll get 56 side effects that were not found in the placebo group.

HOWEVER – if you compare a vaccine to another vaccine or a placebo filled with neurotoxins…..you'll only get a few side effects.

Clever bit of black magic there to pull the wool over literally EVERYONE'S eyes.

Once again….ask your doctor if they knew that vaccines were not tested against true placebos before coming to market. Pretty sure we all know what that answer will be.

On a quick side note – I wanted to dedicate this entire page to simply say one thing:

Follow Del Bigtree and Robert Kennedy Jr's work with the HighWire, the ICAN network, and personally on social media.

These two have done unprecedented things to help bring information to light despite very intense opposition.

I am in no way affiliated with them, I have simply met them and respect them greatly for all the work they've done.

US Vaccine Court

Alright – you ready to wrap this up?

I said I wanted to keep this REALLY simple – which so far I think I've done a pretty good job of.

So OK – we KNOW that vaccines carry risk and can cause harm. They're a medical procedure – and the US Government (well actually YOU the taxpayer...since YOU'RE actually the one that pays for the injuries) has paid out over $4 BILLION dollars in damages since the time vaccine manufacturers were made immune to lawsuits (1986 – Present).

So, what happens if you or someone you know and love is injured by a vaccine?

Well first – you've got to attempt to convince your doctor that vaccines carry risk, and that your child dying within 24 hours of getting 8 vaccines (refer to the graph on page 22 of the Infanrix 6 in 1 vaccine) isn't "coincidence".

THEN have to get them to file a VAERS report – have fun with that.

Then you've got get yourself a lawyer, get all of the documentation, and THEN – you get to go sue the US Government in a special "secret" court where YOU need to PROVE that the vaccine caused injury.

You're not allowed to use the rulings from other cases (as they're closed and secret in regards to the details), you need to understand all the medical terminology, find doctors to come testify on your behalf, and you need to use the studies the DHS has done on vaccines to prove that the vaccine caused your injury.

BUT WAIT!!!

The DHS never did the studies, did they???

I've actually made it FAR less intimidating sounding than it actually is to enter the vaccine court and attempt to win your case – as it's completely loaded to ensure that literally NO ONE gets their case approved, and often times they draw it out as long as they possibly can so parents either A.) Go broke and can't afford to continue or B.) Draw it out for as long as possible so parents eventually just give up and move on with their lives.

DESPITE all of this – over $4 Billion dollars has still been paid out to those injured or killed by vaccines.

COVID-19 Coincidence

As is not only said that "there is no such thing as coincidence" – so too, is it said "intelligence is the ability to notice patterns."

I'd like to point something out, that simply fits with the pattern of what this entire book has been about.

During the COVID19 pLandemic,

There was roughly a 30% drop in deaths of infants under 1 year old.

Adolescent and teen deaths were unchanged, and elderly deaths were up – but magically, the deaths of children under 1 year old were INSTANTLY slashed by 30%.

So when one takes a look and speculates – what are some possible explanations for this?

I personally – don't have many, in fact I have only 1 logical explanation of what could cause this.

The only thing that would have been fairly universal across infants that would cause only their age group to have a drop in death rates THAT significant...

Is that people stopped taking their infants to their pediatricians and getting them vaccinated.

Here is the link to learn more about this data specifically:
https://www.ageofautism.com/2020/06/lessons-from-the-lockdown-a-white-paper-from-health-choice.html

Here's an excellent exercise to partake in as well.

The link above – is NOT exactly what I'd call a "trusted source". It's not an "official agency", nor is it even a "mainstream" article.

This however – is the only reason you're hearing about it.

Just because a website isn't "credible" exactly – doesn't mean that the information they're going to share isn't fully legitimate.

Many times only on "obscure" websites will you find the data that people don't want found.

I mean….all of the points I've brought up in this book, undeniably true (to the 99.9% hopefully at least).

Not ONE of these common sense points have been covered anywhere "official" or "mainstream" – even though they are news-worthy beyond anything that makes its way onto the Tell-Lie-Vision currently.

Whatever the argument, and whatever the source – simply try to see if it is True or not, and use what can be applicable, discard the rest. The revolution is not exactly going to be televised.

I'll be very clear here.

I'm not saying I'm right.

I'm simply pointing something out – that follows the pattern of vaccine injuries NOT being reported and NOT being as rare as we're told.

If you can come up with a better idea than what I and other people have thought – I'm always all ears.

But after reading just an INTRODUCTION to all of the things wrong with our idea of what we THINK vaccines are, and the REALITY of WHAT WE HAVE – to me it is not that insane of an idea to think that hey, perhaps vaccines ARE causing more damage than most people care to think about.

Once again however, I'm not saying believe me.

I'm simply saying give it some thought – and investigate and form the best conclusion you can, but be HONEST with yourself about the things you discover. It's always easiest to lie to ourselves.

Emotional Regret

One thing I'd like to point out – is that if you have already vaccinated your child or children, you're going to have an incredible level of subconscious protection programs running to keep you from acknowledging the reality of the unintended consequences of vaccines that people are not very informed of usually.

This is not to belittle or degrade you in any way – it simply is to ask you to be aware of protection mechanisms that you've installed in your own mind to keep you from looking at things in an honest light. Don't let not wanting something to be true, keep you from admitting what is.

This is NOT shaming I repeat. The thing to realize is – there a MULTIPLE streams of disinformation that are pumped out to the public, unfortunately even through your doctor – that are deliberately there to protect huge levels of profits.

Just be kind to yourself – and do your best to not let yourself get in the way of what is true.

Like I said – I was going to keep this short and simple.

I'm not here as I stated earlier to sit and go into long, drawn out, gigantic scientific debates on the tobacco science we're fed regarding vaccines. As a parent – you honestly probably don't have that kind of time to get up to speed on EVERY single one of the talking points. I mean, heck – this book was pretty much just off the top of my head of SIMPLE points, and it's STILL a lot grasp.

Here's the simplest point I'd like to make:

If these SIMPLE, COMMON SENSE talking points pointing out gigantic FLAWS with the vaccine program – that probably 99% of doctors are unaware of, and an even greater percentage of parents most likely are unaware…

There really isn't any reason a parent even needs to start breaking into the actual science – because we can't even get past the simple, common sense parts without our jaws dropping to the floor.

If the SIMPLE parts are THIS skewed and delusional in regards to common sense, simply imagine how badly the science is twisted (I can assure you – I have spent the time looking into it, and it's JUST as BAD as you can imagine).

Summing it up:

The most dangerous belief you can entertain – is your own opinion.

I don't want anyone to take anything from this book as the "End All Truth on Everything".

This book is far from it.

It is simply here to be a quick read, that highlights the VERY large problems, that you do NOT have to be a doctor or scientist to understand.

These are problems PARENTS can comprehend, and in my opinion, should be ENRAGED over.

Your children are being used as an experiment, and you're paying the price for it.

But these things,

Are just my opinions.

The facts are what they are,

Please spend time coming to your own conclusions.

For those wanting to learn more about vaccines – below is a list of many different people, books, or pages to follow for more information.

Del Bigtree – The HighWire
I share no affiliation with him or his work – I simply love what he does and he does it well.

Robert F Kennedy Jr – Children's Health Defense
Equally as great at dismantling the false narrative as Del

www.icandecide.org
Del and Robert's website for news around vaccine updates

Catie Clobes (Facebook) -
A mother who's child was killed by vaccines and was stonewalled by the medical community at every turn – you literally can't make up the stuff that they've done to her, the greatest warrior mama you've ever encountered in the name of Justice and Truth
#JusticeForEvee
https://www.justiceforevee.org/

Ashley Everley (Facebook) -
A toxicologist who put together one of the best resources ever regarding vaccine science and the flaws.
Download or cruise the collection of her genius at:
https://vaccine.guide/

www.learntherisk.org
A fantastic collection of articles, resources, research, parents rights, and where to get involved.

NVIC.org
A wonderful resource for everything vaccine related, talking points, updates, vaccine bills, and various other needed points

So You're Going To Have A Baby – Amazon and Kindle book
A book I coauthored with a friend for those who wanted a little peek into the science of vaccines – as well as Pitocin, epidurals, ultrasounds, prenatal vitamins,

folic acid vs folate, MTHFR, fluoride, mercury fillings, and nearly anything else you can imagine regarding your pregnancy and navigating the medical world before, during, and after the birth if your baby.

www.stayhealthymyfriends.win

www.ingramcontent.com/pod-product-compliance
Lightning Source LLC
Chambersburg PA
CBHW080922160726
48000CB00009B/3091